Depression & Suicide, the Long View
Your 18th Psychiatric Consultation
William Yee M.D., J.D.
Copyright Applied for 11/30/2020

Suicide, the Big Picture

The evaluation and treatment of depression and suicide is a complex proposition.

The current approach in medicine is to apply the best practice based upon the current available evidence.

Because technology and science is rapidly changing, yesterday's practice is not today's practice.

In medicine there is a tension between the classical approach characterized by Occam's Razor and the modern approach which embraces risk management, and a treatment plan that anticipates multiple trajectories for future change.

Occam's Razor is the old practice of medicine whereby the simplest diagnosis was the preferred diagnosis.

That practice does not embrace false negatives and false positives.

A false negative is when the negative diagnosis is wrong.

A false positive is when a positive diagnosis is wrong.

The best practice in medicine includes the lowest effective dose to minimize medication side effects.

The best practice in medicine includes medication tapers to determine what the lowest effective dose is or even the possibility that the medication is no longer needed when the medication is tapered to no medication.

The best practice in medicine to include the possibility of concurrent medical problems. For example, a low thyroid function precipitating a depression.

The best practice in medicine includes a treatment plan that educates the patient as to what to do when symptoms get worse or medications manifest side effects.

The brain has about one hundred billion neurons with a range of one hundred to one thousand trillion synapses connecting the brain.

I leave it to the reader to fact check the above and all that follows for further consideration, clarification, and correction.

Recent research in the function of the brain has revealed that over the course of every one hundred days there is a thirteen percent change in the fingerprint of the brain.

The fingerprint of the brain is the picture of the brain while active.

That can be construed to mean that each one hundred days of experience alters thirteen percent of the activity of the brain.

Good luck, bad luck, psychotherapy, meditation, medications, and other factors combine to alter thirteen percent of the brain's function every one hundred days,

The remaining eighty seven percent of the brain activity remains stable in regulating sleep, appetite respiration, heart rate, temperature, vision, hearing, proprioception, digestion, sweating, adrenal function, pituitary function, menstrual cycles, touch, smell, and other basic functions.

For fact checking I refer the reader to:

Quantifying Differences and Similarities in Whole-Brain White Matter Architecture Using Local Connectome Fingerprints
Fang-Cheng Yeh ,
Jean M. Vettel,
Aarti Singh,
Barnabas Poczos,
Scott T. Grafton,
Kirk I. Erickson,
Wen-Yih I. Tseng,
Timothy D. Verstynen
Published: November 15, 2016
https://doi.org/10.1371/journal.pcbi.100520
3

See also:
Researchers Develop Way To "Fingerprint" the Brain

New Tool Uncovers How Brain's Structural Connections Are Individually Unique

November 15, 2016

https://www.cmu.edu/dietrich/news/news-stories/2016/november/brain-fingerprint.html
Dietrich College of Humanities and Social Sciences
5000 Forbes Avenue, Pittsburgh, PA 15213
(412) 268-2830
Legal Info www.cmu.edu
The Army Research Laboratory funded this research.

In late adolescence and early adult life the brain is highly active in pruning synapses that are not being used. This allows for the growth of new synapses to allow continued development of skills that are being used.

It is believed that this pruning may be disrupted by inflammation so that there is random pruning, and the brain becomes separated into islands of cells.

This may explain the emergence of anosognosia.

Anosognosia is the failure of a person to recognize a part of his body as part of the person.

Anosognosia is the failure of a person to recognize a memory as a part of the person.

Anosognosia is the failure of a person to recognize a thought, smell, emotion, sensation, or anything else as being a part of that person.

Without that connection the person concludes that the thoughts, memories, emotions, sensations, etc. are inserted by satellites, etc.

Anosognosia is the basis for delusions, hallucinations, and paranoia in schizophrenia and after traumatic brain injuries.

To my knowledge the first time anosognosia was published in the medical literature was over a hundred years ago.

A neurologist published an anecdotal report of a patient who had a head injury. The result of the head injury was that the patient no longer knew his left arm was part of his body.

This was anosognosia caused by brain damage.

As a result, the patient became convinced that the arm belonged to someone else.

The patient cut off that left arm.

There was no discussion of whether the patient experienced pain.

Perhaps he was able to ignore the pain due to anosognosia for the pain, the belief that the pain was the pain of another person.

This may lead to an alternative to opioids for chronic pain.

It is believed that this may be the root cause of schizophrenia which most commonly emerges in late adolescence and early adult life, a time of very active pruning.

Anosognosia is very common in schizophrenia.

Anosognosia is probably the root cause of hallucinations, delusions, and paranoia regarding voices, visual images, memories, pain, heat, cold.

Anosognosia is probably the root cause of the belief that friends, and relatives are imposters who have replaced friends and relatives. The belief that people are imposters is called Capgras Syndrome.

The pruning of synapses in the schizophrenic brain results in isolation of islands of cells that continue to function, but are no longer perceived as part of one self.

For fact checking and a deeper look, I refer the reader to:

Increased synapse elimination by microglia in schizophrenia patient-derived models of synaptic pruning. Carl M. Sellgren, Jessica Gracias, Bradley Watmuff, Jonathan D. Biag, Jessica M. Thanos, Paul B. Whittredge, Ting Fu, Kathleen Worringer, Hannah E. Brown, Jennifer Wang, Ajamete Kaykas, Rakesh Karmacharya, Carleton P. Goold, Steven D. Sheridan, Roy H. Perlis. Nature

Neuroscience, 2019; DOI: 10.1038/s41593-018-0334-7

Glial cells are central to the pruning process, which is a lifelong process and responsible for the 13% change in the brain fingerprint every one hundred days.

Glial cells are now believed to be active in the function of the brain despite their lack of synapses.

Glial cells partner with neurons to process memories, partner with the immune system to fight infections, partner with DNA to promote brain development, It is believed that glial cells partner with neurons and the pituitary gland's endocrine system to participate in all functions of the brain.

I refer the reader to the following for a fact check and entry into this topic:

Glial Brain Cells, Long in Neurons' Shadow, Reveal Hidden Powers
Elena Renken
Contributing Writer
ABSTRACTIONS BLOG

Suicide often occurs with the first episode of schizophrenia and should be considered in every psychotic break, especially in late adolescence and early adult life.

This fact impacts the military as this is the age group most heavily recruited.

Although there is remarkable progress in the diagnosis and treatment of mental illness, it remains very difficult to diagnose and treat suicidal episodes.

The first reason is the complexity of the human brain and the fact that the available tools are primitive and crude in comparison to the complexity and sophistication of the brain.

For example, the prediction of suicide is less accurate than the flip of a coin.

The reason is that it is easy to explain the suicide in retrospect, it is not easy to predict the suicide before it happens. As a result, suicide is over diagnosed to avoid an error that cannot be corrected.

Diagnosing a suicide that does not happen affords an opportunity for corrective action.

Failing to diagnose a suicide that does happen does not allow for a corrective action.

For a detailed analysis and bibliography, I refer the reader to:
The role of prediction in suicide prevention
Matthew Michael Large, BSc, MBBS, FRANZCP, DMedSci
Dialogues Clin Neurosci. 2018 Sep; 20(3): 197–205.
doi: 10.31887/DCNS.2018.20.3/mlarge
PMCID: PMC6296389
PMID: 30581289

The diagnosis of suicide is followed by managing the risk and treating the stress, anxiety, and depression that generate the suicidal episode.

The suicidal episode can be generated by cultural demands for ritual suicide to preserve the honor of the individual and family.

Seppuku, also known as hara-kiri, is a Japanese example of ritual suicide.

"He bought the farm," is a military phrase from the nineteen fifties that referred to a deadly plane crash. It reflected the wishes of many airmen to stop flying, return to the states, buy a farm and live peacefully ever after.

During the Great Depression many farmers committed suicide. Some may have done it so their families could collect life insurance and pay for the farm

There may be grief, depression and other aspects of mental illness present. However, the cultural basis for suicide is not a product of mental illness as mental illness is understood in Western culture.

Now there is physician assisted suicide, which expands the breadth and complexity of diagnosis and treatment of suicide. If the patient has suicidal thoughts, should the physician offer assisted suicide?

For a fact check and entry into this topic, I refer the reader to:

Physician-Assisted Suicide and Euthanasia in Washington State Patient Requests and Physician Responses
Anthony L. Back, MD; Jeffrey I. Wallace, MD, MPH; Helene E. Starks, MPH; et alRobert A. Pearlman, MD, MPH
JAMA. 1996;275(12):919-925.
doi:10.1001/jama.1996.03530360029034

The patient should be educated as to the fact that the convention is to make a formal diagnosis of mental illness only if there is impairment in a major life function.

The patient will carry that diagnosis and record of impairment for life.

This is not trivial, as it affects employability.

Doctors and other health care professionals risk loss of medical licensure, loss of hospital privileges and loss of malpractice insurance if they have committed a crime or are impaired by mental illness.

In the military the service member must maintain a high level of physical and mental functioning at all times.

Impairment by mental illness or the treatment of mental illness is a reason for a medical discharge.

A medication such as Ambien, Oxycontin, Xanax, Prazosin, Elavil, or Thorazine may sedate a patient enough to give rise to a ticket for driving impaired. If there are children in the car, Child Protective Services may be called.

The patient may take the medication and lose a driver's license and have the patient's children placed into foster care for safety reasons.

Military service members are required to maintain a higher average level of physical, mental and emotional functioning than the average civilian.

This is in the face of multiple deployments and separations from family, friends and country.

The assertion that a health care worker or military service member is not stable, paranoid or impulsive is a serious matter not to be ignored.

It is important to be careful and specific in assessments and the service member and other subjects should be given every opportunity to make the record complete according to their knowledge and understanding.

The notion of, "State Bound Learning," needs to be examined for a better understanding of behavior during episodes of mental illness.

State bound learning is learning associated with different emotional states. This explains how a person with PTSD can abruptly change from calm to agitated and out of control.

This also can explain the phenomenon of, "Dissociative Personality Disorder."

I refer the reader to the following articles for a fact check and introduction to this topic:

State-dependent memory
From Wikipedia, the free encyclopedia

The Influences of Emotion on Learning and Memory
Chai M. Tyng, Hafeez U. Amin, Mohamad N. M. Saad, and Aamir S. Malik
Front Psychol. 2017; 8: 1454.
Published online 2017 Aug 24. doi: 10.3389/fpsyg.2017.01454
PMCID: PMC5573739, PMID: 28883804

The Long View

I have been practicing psychiatry without interruption since 1972 in Michigan, Indian, Kentucky, California, and Texas. I am board certified in psychiatry.

In 1970 I was doing a rotation in surgery at the Detroit General Hospital in Detroit, Michigan.

The surgery rotation had Friday Morbidity and Mortality rounds.

All the surgeries resulting in death and complications were examined.

The purpose was to identify the cause of the death and complications.

After the cause of the death and complications were determined there was a discussion to determine all possible alternative treatments.

Then there was a discussion as to what the best alternative was.

The best alternative became the new standard of practice for all future patients.

This discussion did not involve blame or punitive actions.

The only action was determining the best practice and making the best practice future practice.

I call this process error trapping and corrective action.

Error trapping and corrective action has been part of every interaction that I have with a patient since that time.

I apply the best practice that I know of with each transaction.

If there is a bad result, I identify all possible treatment alternatives and then I identify the best practice among them.

That best practice becomes part of all my future practices.

From time to time, I research literature on a topic such as the diagnosis and treatment of suicide.

I identify the best practices and they become part of all my future practices.

I have a template for evaluating and treating patients.

That template is like the flight check that a pilot uses.

It has all the best practices built in so that I do not forget an important practice.

That template changes with each patient.

That template has served me well in regard to minimizing errors.

That template has allowed me to survive the past fifty years of peer review as a medical student and practicing physician.

I have practiced as an emergency room physician in 1973 and 1974 at Detroit General Hospital in Detroit, Michigan.

I practiced psychiatry at Henry Ford Hospital in Detroit and taught medical students and residents in psychiatry.

I have been the medical director of two mental health centers in Indiana for about twelve years.

I have been the Chairman of the Department of Psychiatry in a community hospital in Michigan.

I have worked in three state Forensic Psychiatric Hospitals in Michigan and California.

I have worked in regional hospitals in Michigan, Kentucky and California with busy emergency rooms.

I have worked in prisons in Michigan and California.

All these places addressed suicide with formal policies of suicide precautions including physical restraints and court ordered medications.

All these facilities experienced patient suicides despite extensive written policies, procedures, and practices reviewed by the joint commission and hospital administration.

In the 1970's there was a literature regarding the fact that antidepressants increased energy before there was a subjective reduction in depression.

The result was the literature reported successful suicides shortly after the start antidepressant medications.

I refer the reader to the following article for fact checking and an introduction to the topic:

Do Antidepressants Increase Suicide Attempts? Do They Have Other Risks?
Madeline Levin, MPH, Nicolas J. Jury, PhD, Kousha Mohseni, MS, Varuna Srinivasan, MBBS MPH,
National Center for Health Research
1001 Connecticut Avenue NW, Suite 1100
Washington, DC 20036
(202) 223-4000
©2020. All rights reserved.

Medications for depression have black box warnings about possible suicide.

I refer the reader to the FDA labels for all the antidepressants which state in principle:

"Suicidality and Antidepressant Drugs Antidepressants increased the risk compared to placebo of suicidal thinking and behavior (suicidality) in children, adolescents, and young adults in short-term studies of major depressive disorder (MDD) and other psychiatric disorders."

Prescribing antidepressant medication does not resolve the risk of suicide.

If there are suicidal thoughts, there needs to be a comprehensive assessment of the risk factors and protective factors and a plan for safety.

The safety plan needs to be individualized according to the patient's history and circumstances and clinical presentation.

The safety plan will change as the clinical presentation and circumstances change.

If antidepressants cause a temporary spike in suicide while the energy is increased but the depression has not been resolved, are there additional medications?

It can take two to twelve weeks for the antidepressants to have a significant effect on depression.

ECT is considered an effective intervention. However, many patients

during the first twelve weeks of treatment
with antidepressants.

Benzodiazepines and Ambien increase the
risk of suicide.

I refer the reader to the following for
more details and a bibliography:

Hypnotic hazards: adverse effects of
zolpidem and other z-drugs
LG Olson
Aust Prescr 2008;31:146-9
1 December 2008
DOI: 10.18773/austprescr.2008.084

and
Association between benzodiazepines and
suicide risk: a matched case-control
study.
Cato, V., Holländare, F., Nordenskjöld, A.
et al.
BMC Psychiatry 19, 317 (2019).
https://doi.org/10.1186/s12888-019-2312-3

and
Benzodiazepines are Contraindicated in
Post Traumatic Stress Disorder (PTSD)
by Sonja Styblo, MSW | Sep 10, 2016

and
Benzodiazepines, Health Care Utilization, and Suicidal Behavior in Veterans With Posttraumatic Stress Disorder
Rishi Deka, PhD; Craig J. Bryan, PsyD, ABPP; Joanne LaFleur, PharmD; Gary Oderda, PharmD; Abril Atherton, PharmD; and Vanessa Stevens, PhD
J Clin Psychiatry 2018;79(6):17m12038
https://doi.org/10.4088/JCP.17m12038

There are anecdotal case reports of hydroxyzine associated with suicide.

Most of the suicides with hydroxyzine were associated with multiple other psychotropic medications.

One interpretation is that hydroxyzine does not protect patient from suicide associated with other psychotropic medications.

A second interpretation is that hydroxyzine can cause suicide in the presence of other psychotropic medications.

A third interpretation is that hydroxyzine is unpredictable in the presence of other psychotropic medications.

In general, the best practice is the lowest effective dose of medications.

Also, monotherapy is preferable to polypharmacy with psychotropic medications.

Being on multiple psychotropic medications is not considered the best practice in psychiatry.

Hydroxyzine is often prescribed with multiple other psychotropic medications that clouds the issue of suicidality and the cause of a successful suicide.

Review the following article for a fact check;

A Fatal Case Involving Hydroxyzine
G.R. Johnson

Journal of Analytical Toxicology, Volume 6, Issue 2, March-April 1982, Pages 69–70, https://doi.org/10.1093/jat/6.2.69

There is literature on the use of psychostimulants for use with antidepressants.

The primary use for psychostimulants is for ADHD.

I refer the reader to:

Methamphetamine use can cause deficits in memory, executive functions, information processing speed, motor skills, language, and visuoconstructional abilities. Methamphetamine can cause frontostriatal neurotoxicity.

I refer the reader to:
Neurocognitive Effects of Methamphetamine: A Critical Review and Meta-analysis
J. Cobb Scott, Steven Paul Woods, Georg E. Matt, Rachel A. Meyer, Robert K. Heaton, J. Hampton Atkinson & Igor Grant

Neuropsychology Review volume 17, pages275–297(2007)

and
Role of Dopamine Receptors in ADHD: A Systematic Meta-analysis
Jing Wu, Haifan Xiao, Hongjuan Sun, Li Zou & Ling-Qiang Zhu
Molecular Neurobiology volume 45, pages605–620(2012)

and
ADHD in Adults and Its Relation with Methamphetamine Use: National Data
Meelie Bordoloi, Geetha Chandrashekar & Naveen Yarasi
Current Developmental Disorders Reports volume 6, pages224–227(2019).

The FDA Label for Adderall warns against addiction and sudden death.

The FDA Label clearly states that impairment in functioning is a requirement.

The FDA Label for Adderall warns the patient about, "psychotic episodes at recommended doses, overstimulation, restlessness, irritability, euphoria, dyskinesia, dysphoria, depression, tremor, tics, aggression, anger, logorrhea, dermatillomania."

People with ADHD are more likely to have accidents.

Serious transport accidents in adults with ADHD, and the effect of medication: A population based study
Zheng Chang, MSc,1, Paul Lichtenstein, PhD, Brian M. D'Onofrio, PhD, Arvid Sjölander, PhD, and Henrik Larsson, PhD
JAMA Psychiatry. 2014 Mar 1; 71(3): 319–325.
doi: 10.1001/jamapsychiatry.2013.4174
PMCID: PMC3949159
NIHMSID: NIHMS532652
PMID: 24477798

Antipsychotics may be used for dissociative behaviors, anger, aggression, disorganized behaviors, and explosiveness associated with PTSD,

I refer the reader to:
Use of Antipsychotics in the Treatment of Post-Traumatic Stress Disorder

Babatunde Adetunji, MD, Maju Mathews, MD, Adedapo Williams, MD, Kumar Budur, MD, Manu Mathews, MD, Jamal Mahmud, MD, and Thomas Osinowo, MD
Psychiatry (Edgmont). 2005 Apr; 2(4): 43–47.
Published online 2005 Apr.
PMCID: PMC3004738
PMID: 21179651

Every patient that has a suicidal thought cannot be admitted to a psychiatric hospital because there are not enough available beds.

I have worked in an emergency room as an emergency room physician, and I have consulted as a psychiatrist in many emergency rooms.

My experience is that most suicide attempts are treated in the emergency room and released home for outpatient treatment.

In 2018 526,000 adults were admitted to a psychiatric hospital after a suicide attempt.

In 2019 there were 1.4 million suicide attempts among adults.

This information is very difficult to obtain as there is no formal mandatory reporting to allow all the data to be collected and reviewed.

I refer the reader to:

Suicide-related hospitalizations among adults in the U.S. 2013-2019
Published by John Elflein, Sep 18, 2020

It is a curious fact, but a fact. Patients who are forced into a psychiatric hospital admission are more likely to attempt suicide after discharge.

Fact check the following:

Perceived Coercion During Admission Into Psychiatric Hospitalization Increases Risk of Suicide Attempts After Discharge
Joshua T. Jordan PhD Dale E. McNiel PhD
First published: 04 June 2019
https://doi.org/10.1111/sltb.12560

The United States Department of Defense is heavily invested in the prevention of suicide among members of the military.

I refer the reader to the following:

VA/DoD CLINICAL PRACTICE GUIDELINE FOR ASSESSMENT AND MANAGEMENT OF PATIENTS AT RISK FOR SUICIDE Department of Veterans Affairs Department of Defense Prepared by: The Assessment and Management of Risk for Suicide Working Group With support from: The Office of Quality Safety and Value, VA, Washington, DC & Quality Management Division, United States Army MEDCOM Version 1.0 – June 2013

Ketamine is touted as a rapid and effective intervention tor depression. It is expensive and not widely available.

I refer the reader to the following for a fact check and introduction to the literature:

Efficacy of ketamine therapy in the treatment of depression

Suprio Mandal, Vinod Kumar Sinha, and Nishant Goyal

Indian J Psychiatry. 2019 Sep-Oct; 61(5): 480–485.
doi:10.4103/psychiatry.IndianJPsychiatry_484_18
PMCID: PMC6767816 PMID: 31579184

It is my practice to admit patients to a psychiatric hospital when they are severely depressed and when they have a plan, and an intent, and the means to commit suicide.

Most patients with suicidal thoughts have anxiety and depression that is moderate to severe.

Most patients with suicidal thoughts do not have the plan or intent or means to attempt suicide and are safely treated as outpatients.

I usually offer Lexapro for depression, anxiety and anergy.

I usually offer Remeron for depression, anxiety and insomnia.

If there are suicidal thoughts, I usually offer fifty milligrams of chlorpromazine at bedtime.

Chlorpromazine is effective for bipolar mood swings and mania, anxiety, agitation, aggression, paranoia, hallucinations, porphyria induced psychosis, and aggression associated with conduct disorders

Chlorpromazine does not cause dissociative states or confusion that is associated with Ambien and benzodiazepines like Xanax.

Short-term effects of Chlorpromazine include sedation that requires caution with driving and dangerous machinery. There is the risk al allergy with any drug including Chlorpromazine. There is dry mouth, constipation, and weight gain.

Generally, I do not prescribe the Chlorpromazine for longer than twelve weeks, so long-term side effects are not a consideration.

Chlorpromazine does not prolong the QTc interval as much as Haldol and is much safer than Haldol and other medications.

Aripiprazole and other third generation antipsychotics are stimulating and likely to increase gambling and other impulsive behaviors including suicide for the short term.

I educate the patient and offer the Lexapro and Chlorpromazine. It is always the patient's choice.

The patient is the team leader, and the treatment choices and plan are a collaboration with the patient, and any family or significant other the patient wishes to be part of the treatment team.

A final note regarding scientific research.

There is a crisis in the ability to replicate scientific research.

The issue is that so much research cannot be reproduced.

I refer the reader to two excellent presentations on YouTube:
Is Most Published Research Wrong?
https://www.youtube.com/watch?v=42QuX LucH3Q&t=1s

The Reproducibility Crisis
https://www.youtube.com/watch?v=v778sv ukrtU&list=PLaab1PTCu-Tb1ZmllaDrP4LeL2B12-io3&index=1&t=578s

Summary

I recommend aerobic exercise, meditation and psychotherapy for depression as a first choice.

I recommend antidepressants for depression as a last choice.

Suicidal thoughts change the equation so that antidepressants such as Lexapro or Remeron become an immediate consideration.

Patients that are suicidal are impaired.

Patients that require treatment for ADHD are impaired by impulsive behavior including accidents. They are not appropriate for depressed, suicidal patients.

Antidepressants increase the risk of suicide during the first six to twelve weeks when energy increases before depression decreases.

Psychostimulants increase addiction and suicide risk.

ECT can be used as an emergency treatment of severe depression.

Ketamine may be an emergency treatment.

Thorazine can prevent suicide during the period when antidepressants are stimulating before the depression remits.

Psychotropic medications have hundreds of side effects and impair ability to function upon first exposure until the patient's physiology establishes a new baseline equilibrium regarding stimulation, sleep cycles, eating and other physiologic functions.

Caution in driving, operation of dangerous machinery and chaperoning with childcare and dependent adult care should be given consideration.

The risks of citations for driving while impaired and the potential for child protective services interventions should be considered as part of the patient's decision to take psychotropic medications.

I leave it to the readers to find a psychiatrist that they can trust.
Although I have been doing my best since 1972, I cannot state with certainty that my help is as good or better than any other psychiatrist.
Thank you for your time and attention.
William R. Yee, M.D., J.D.
Board Certified Psychiatrist
Practicing psychiatry without interruption in Michigan, Indiana,

Kentucky, California and Texas since 1972.

At your service.

I am here to do no harm and help if I can.

"Preexisting text," includes names of symptoms, medical illnesses, medications, people, corporations, law cases, statutes, text of statutes, the titles of articles, of books, the content of articles and books cited.
My copyright claim is a clam to the "original text," which is my personal experiences as described in the text above and my commentary on the names of symptoms, medical illnesses, medications, people, corporations, law cases, statues, text of statutes, the titles of articles, of books, the content of articles and books cited.

www.ingramcontent.com/pod-product-compliance
Lightning Source LLC
Chambersburg PA
CBHW021941170526
45157CB00005B/2376